AF207096

# TEENS DEALING WITH
# ADDICTION

by Tammy Gagne

BrightPoint Press

San Diego, CA

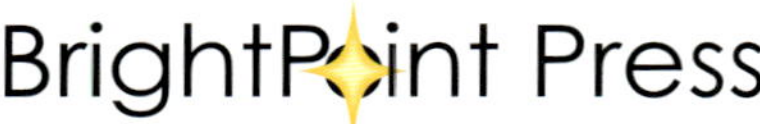

© 2025 BrightPoint Press
an imprint of ReferencePoint Press, Inc.
Printed in the United States

For more information, contact:
BrightPoint Press
PO Box 27779
San Diego, CA 92198
www.BrightPointPress.com



Content Consultant: Jonathan J. Hammersley, PhD, Professor of Psychology, Western Illinois University

LIBRARY OF CONGRESS CATALOGING-IN-PUBLICATION DATA

Name: Gagne, Tammy, author.
Title: Teens Dealing with Addiction / by Tammy Gagne.
Description: San Diego, CA: ReferencePoint Press, Inc., 2025 | Series: Teens Dealing with Adversity | Audience: Grade 6 to 12 | Includes bibliographical references and index.
Identifiers: ISBN: 9781678208868 (hardcover) | ISBN: 9781678208875 (eBook)
The complete Library of Congress record is available at www.loc.gov.

# CONTENTS


**AT A GLANCE**     4

**INTRODUCTION**     6
ADDICTED TO VAPING

**CHAPTER ONE**     12
WHAT IS ADDICTION?

**CHAPTER TWO**     26
HOW ADDICTION AFFECTS TEENS

**CHAPTER THREE**     42
FINDING SUPPORT FOR ADDICTION

Glossary     58
Source Notes     59
For Further Research     60
Index     62
Image Credits     63
About the Author     64

# AT A GLANCE

- Addiction is a disorder in which people feel the need to keep doing a certain activity, even if it harms them.

- Addiction is common among teens. Many young people have substance or behavioral addictions.

- Teens can be addicted to drugs such as nicotine, alcohol, or marijuana. They may also be addicted to behaviors such as gambling.

- People dealing with mental disorders are more likely to develop addictions than their peers.

- Addictions put people at higher risk for health problems, including mental illness, cancer, and even death.

- A person's social life, education, and finances are likely to suffer as a result of addiction.

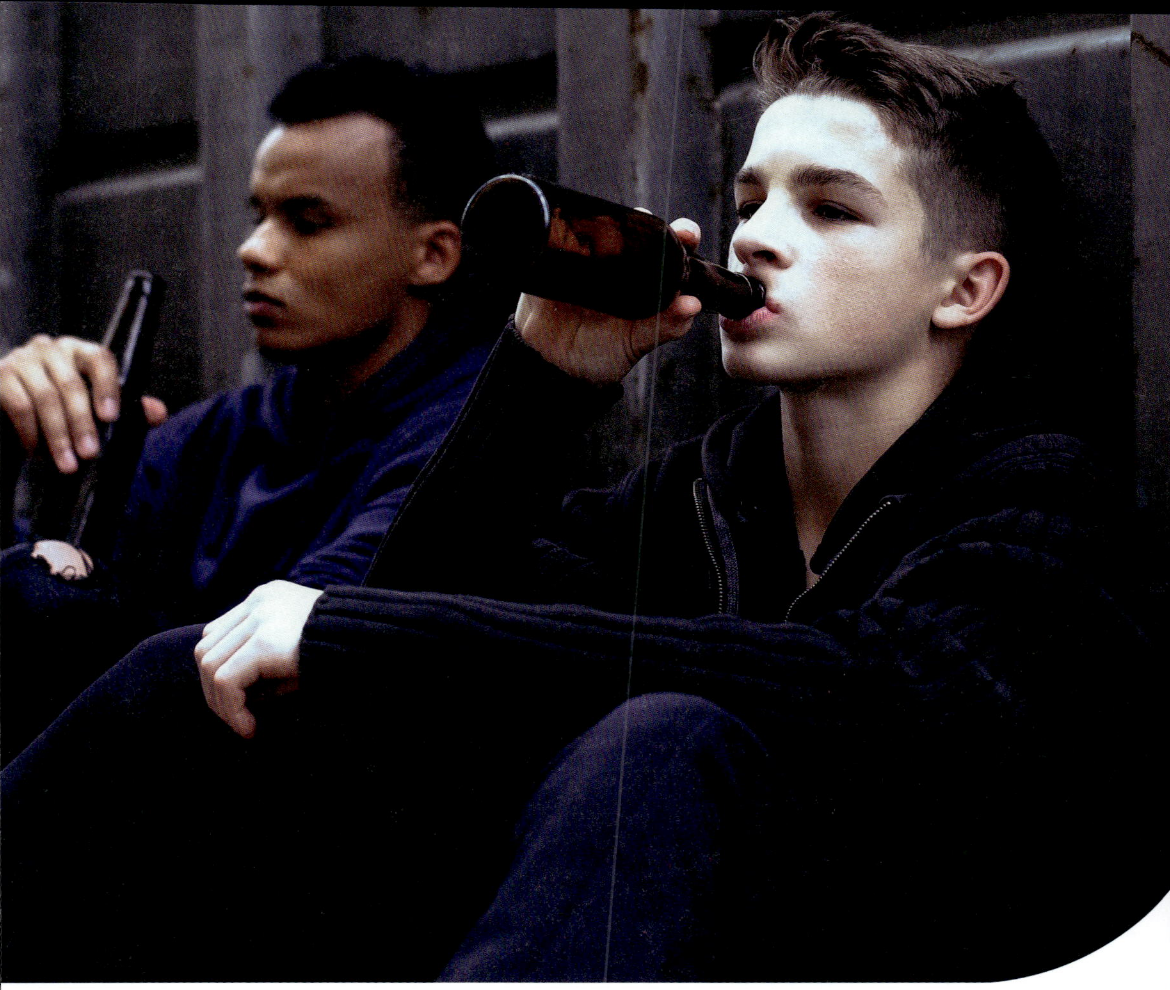

- Many people with addictions do not realize they have a problem until something serious happens.

- People can find support by reaching out to loved ones, seeing a therapist, or speaking to a doctor.

- Treatment centers, medication, and therapy can help people with addiction reclaim their lives.

# ADDICTED TO VAPING

Luka Kinard never expected to become addicted to **vaping**. He was in his first year of high school when his friends pressured him to try it. He finally did. Soon, Luka was vaping all the time. The effects caught up with him quickly. He had been friendly. But vaping made him feel lonely and anxious. He had angry outbursts at home.

In 2023, 33.5 percent of twelfth graders reported that they had used electronic cigarettes at least once in their lives.

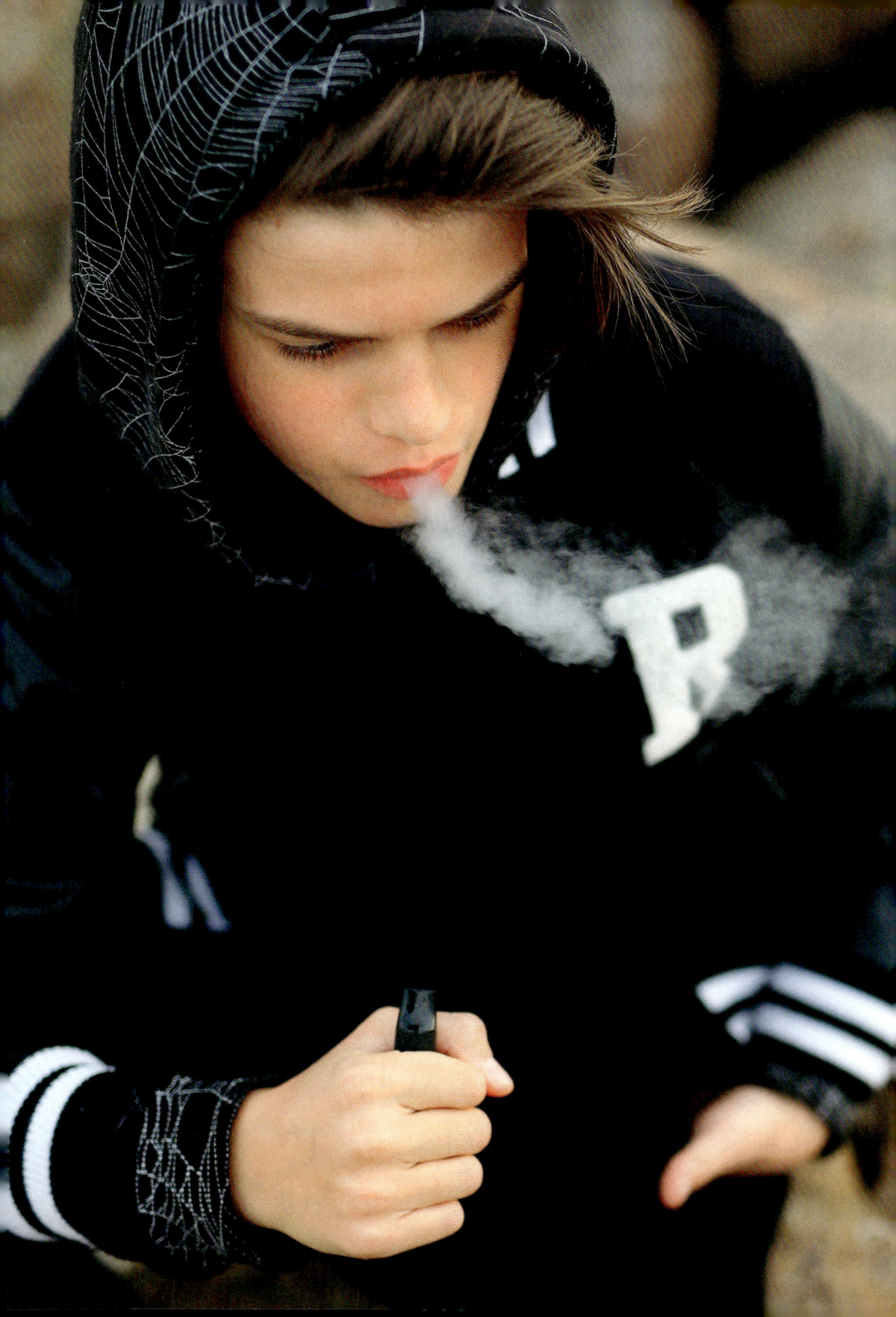

Vaping also affected Luka's physical health. He started losing weight. He began having chest pain and **tremors**. He had cold sweats. "I was actually so freaked out that I was looking up signs of an early heart attack," Luka says. "But I didn't think it was related to the vaping. I didn't want to believe that because that would have been a reason for me to stop."[1]

Vaping started to affect even more parts of his life. He started failing classes. He quit playing sports. He stopped attending Boy Scout meetings.

Luka's parents eventually discovered his addiction. They wanted to help him stop vaping. They sent him to a recovery center. He spent 39 days there. He learned to manage his addiction. Luka has not

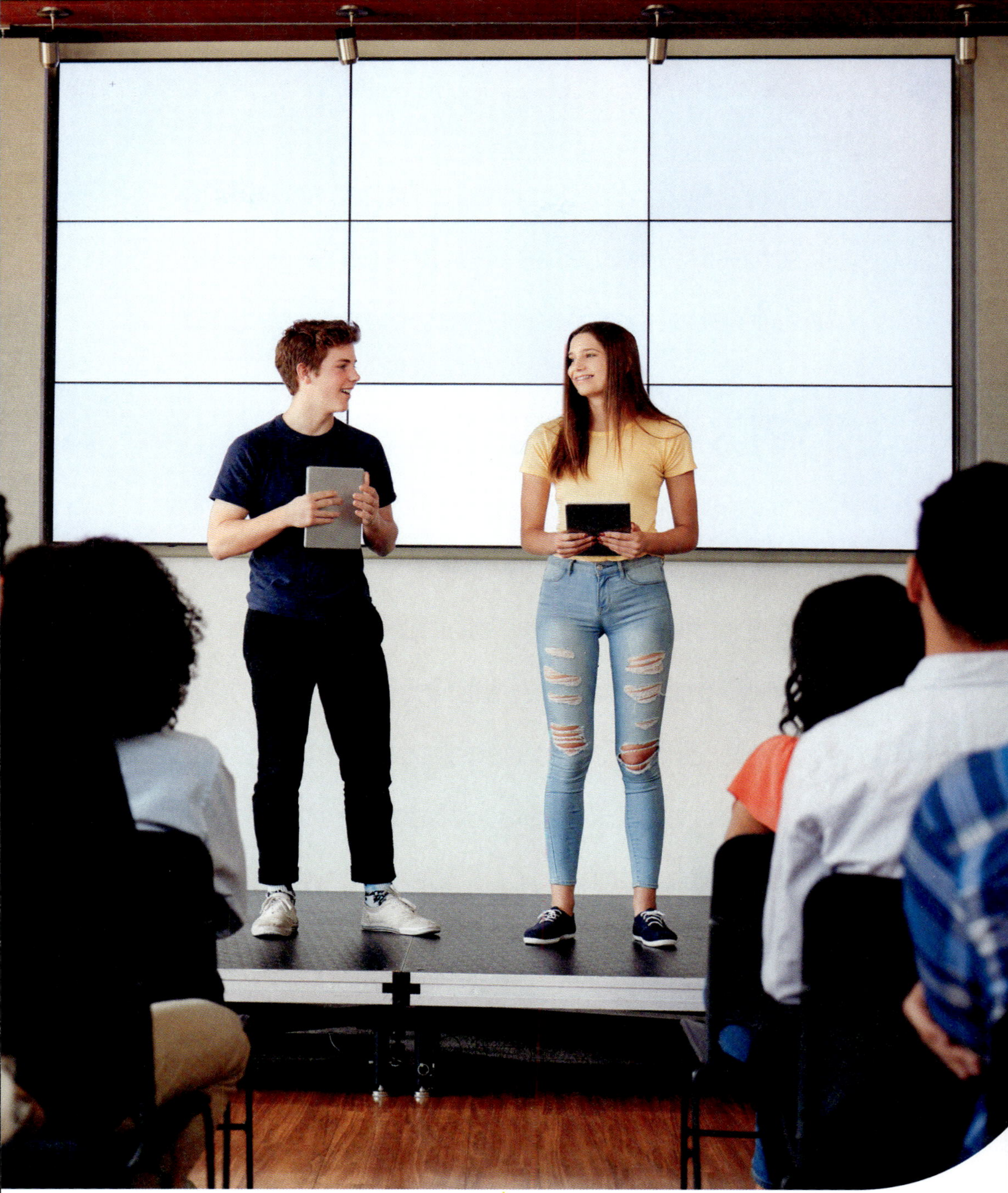

Young people can help teach their peers about the dangers of nicotine use.

vaped since. He decided to start speaking at schools. He wants to warn other young people about the dangers of vaping.

## TYPES OF ADDICTION

Vaping is a common addiction among teens. An addiction is when someone feels the need to keep doing something. Vaping is not the only addiction that teens struggle with. Teens can become addicted to other drugs. It is also possible to become addicted to behaviors. These behaviors include gambling.

Addictions can make it difficult for a person to keep a job or do well in school. They can also damage relationships with friends and family. Some addictions can destroy a person's health.

People with addictions often feel powerless to stop their behavior. But mental health professionals can help. They can provide support. They can also recommend treatment plans. This support can help people with addictions reclaim their lives.

**Support groups, therapy, and help from friends and family give people the tools they need to fight addiction.**

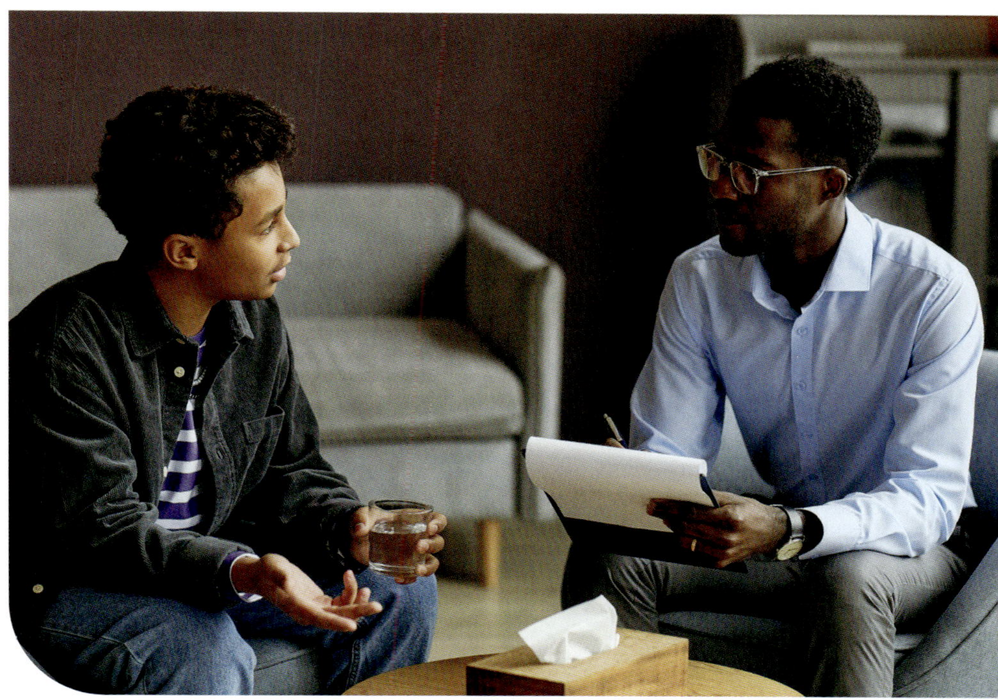

# WHAT IS ADDICTION?

Addiction is a disorder. People with an addiction feel the need to keep doing a certain activity, even if it harms them. Nearly 21 million people in the United States have some type of addiction.

Drug addiction is among the most common addictions for teens. Regular use of alcohol or marijuana can lead to addiction. Other drugs can cause addiction too.

**Alcohol is the most commonly abused drug among teens.**

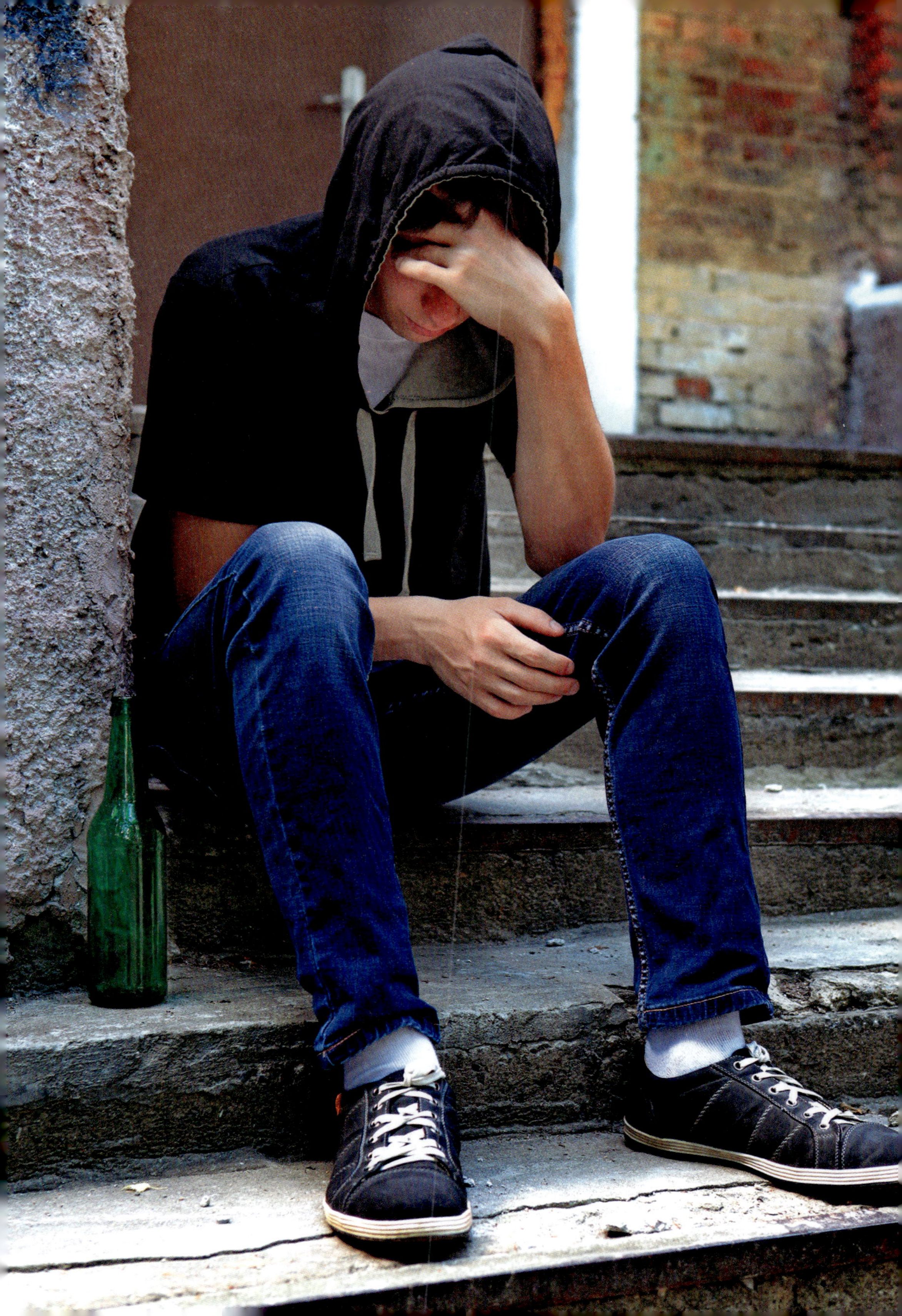

Drug use can seem exciting at first. Drugs can make people feel good physically. They can also make people feel happy or relaxed. A person may continue using a drug to experience those feelings again. A person might also keep using a drug to avoid feeling bad. People may start to crave the feeling that drugs give them. This can lead to addiction.

People can also become addicted to behaviors. Gambling is one such behavior. People who gamble spend money to play games of chance. This can be exciting. The excitement can make people feel good. People can become dependent on these feelings. This can lead to addiction.

It is against the law for people under 21 to smoke cigarettes or use alcohol.

# TWELFTH-GRADE STUDENTS' DRUG USE

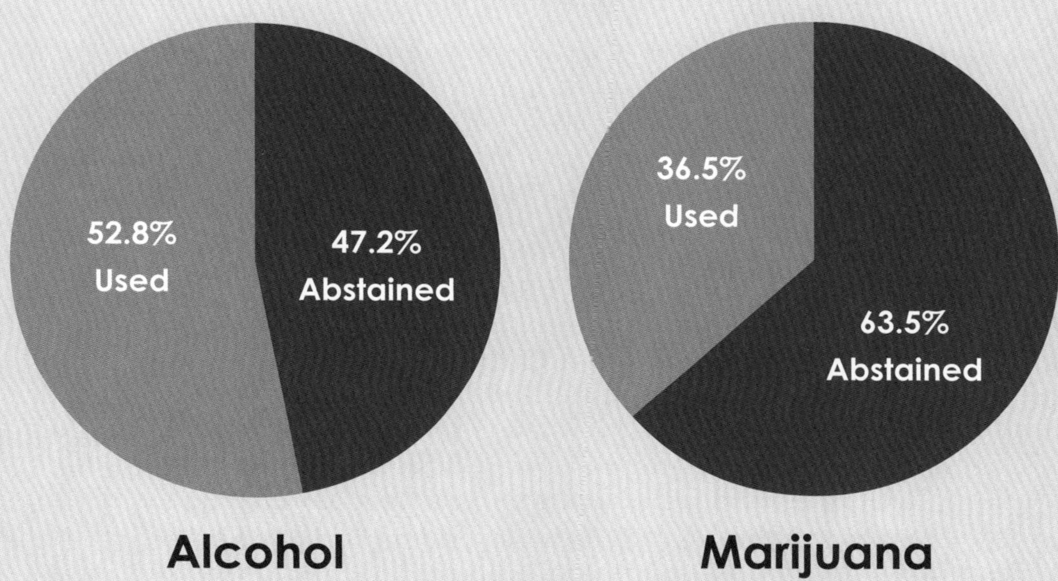


*Source: R.A. Miech, L.D. Johnston, M.E. Patrick, P.M. O'Malley, and J.G. Bachman. "Monitoring the Future National Survey Results on Drug Use, 1975–2023," Monitoring the Future, 2024. https://monitoringthefuture.org.*

**The University of Michigan conducts annual surveys about teen substance use. This graph shows the percentage of twelfth-grade students in 2023 who had ever used alcohol or marijuana.**

But many teens use these drugs anyway.

In 2023, more than 21 percent of eighth graders said they had used illegal drugs.

Twenty-three percent of eighth graders said they had used alcohol.

## HOW ADDICTION HAPPENS

Addiction is a complex disorder. It involves a powerful circuit in the brain known as the reward system. The reward system

**Serotonin and dopamine are two of the many chemicals created by the brain. Both make people feel good and have similar chemical makeups.**

Serotonin

Dopamine

releases chemicals when people do certain behaviors. These chemicals make people feel good. One such chemical is **dopamine**. The reward system teaches people that doing certain behaviors will make them feel good. This encourages them to keep doing the behaviors.

Many important behaviors are reinforced by the brain's reward system. Eating is one such behavior. The reward system releases powerful chemicals when a person eats. The chemicals make the person feel good. This can encourage people to eat again.

The brain's reward system can reinforce other behaviors too. Drinking alcohol triggers a dopamine release that makes a person feel good. Other drugs such as **cocaine** also produce dopamine releases.

Many seemingly harmless activities can trigger the reward system. Gaming is one such behavior. Dr. David Greenfield is the founder of the Center for Internet and Technology Addiction. He says, "Playing video games floods the pleasure center of the brain with dopamine."[2] Some game designers make games just challenging enough to let players feel accomplished.

## Tolerance

Addictions get stronger over time. People's bodies get used to dopamine. This effect is called tolerance. People who develop a tolerance need to increase their usage to get the same level of pleasure as they did in the past. People addicted to alcohol may need to drink more. People addicted to gambling may need to make bigger bets.

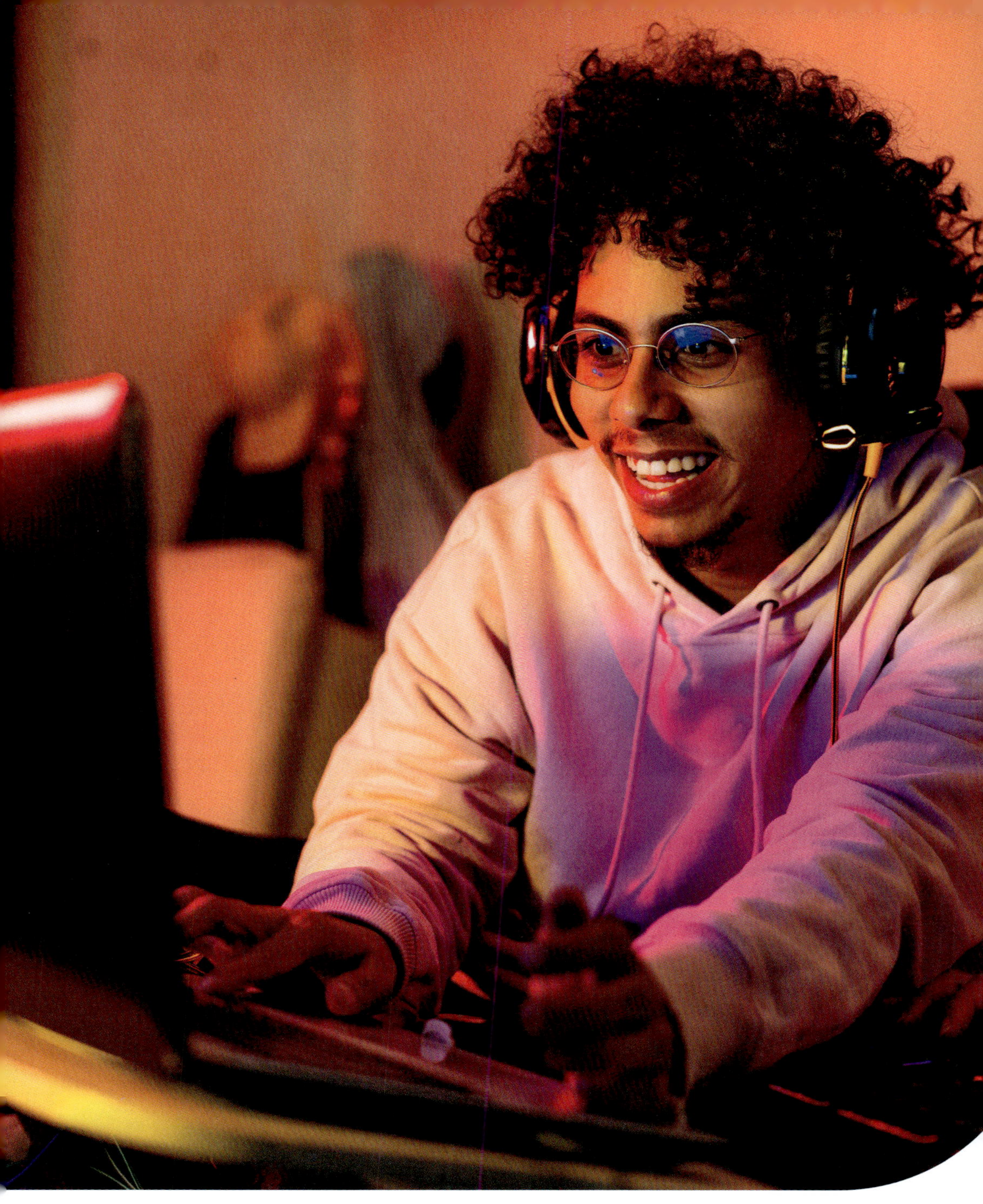

Some doctors believe people can become addicted to video gaming or internet usage.

They reward people for spending time or money on the game. This encourages people to keep gaming. This can eventually lead to addictive behavior.

The object of an addiction becomes more important to people with each use. Soon, other activities become less important. Even things that once brought people joy may no longer hold their interest. They may have trouble focusing on anything but their addiction.

It can be hard to tell when a person develops an addiction. But there are three symptoms that people can look for. The first is engaging with the object of addiction even when there are negative consequences. The second is craving the object of addiction. The third is feeling a

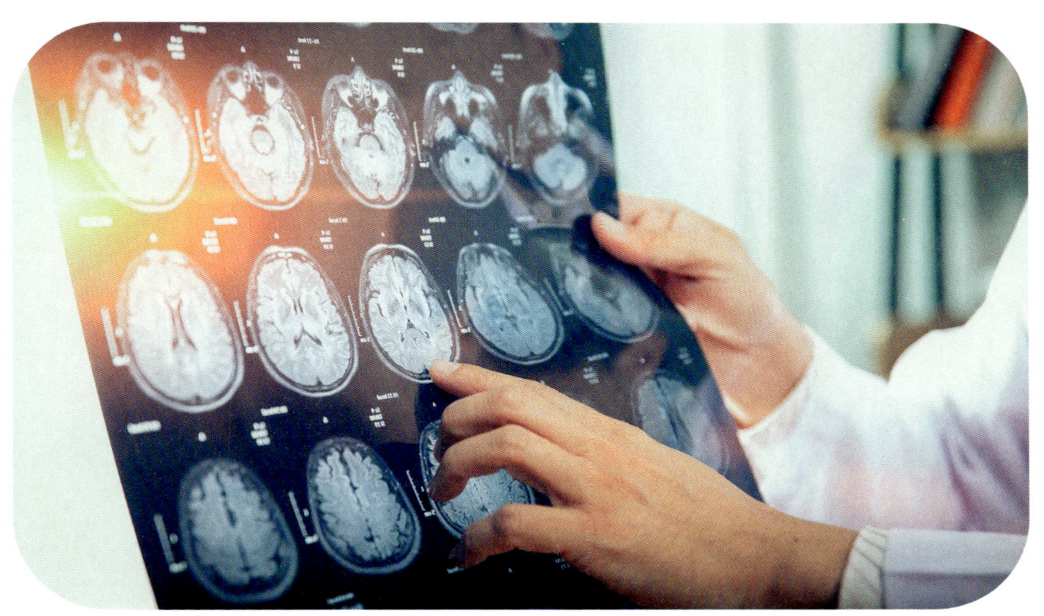

**The brain finishes developing in a person's mid to late 20s.**

loss of control when engaging with the object of addiction.

## HIGHER ADDICTION RISKS

Teens have developing brains. This makes them more likely to form addictions than older adults. Young people also develop addictions faster than adults. Jeanette Friedman is a social worker. She helps young people with addictions. She says,

"If you start drinking at 30, you don't get addicted nearly as fast as if you start drinking at 15."[3]

Teens are also more likely to develop behavioral addictions. Rates of gambling addiction are between two and four times higher for teenagers than for adults. Experts think this may be because young people have less impulse control. Dr. Timothy Fong works for the UCLA Gambling Studies Program. He says,

> *"Young people are significantly at higher risk of developing gambling disorder than adults, in part because their brains are not fully developed. Their ability to evaluate risk [and] their ability to handle loss [aren't] as secure as an adult."[4]*

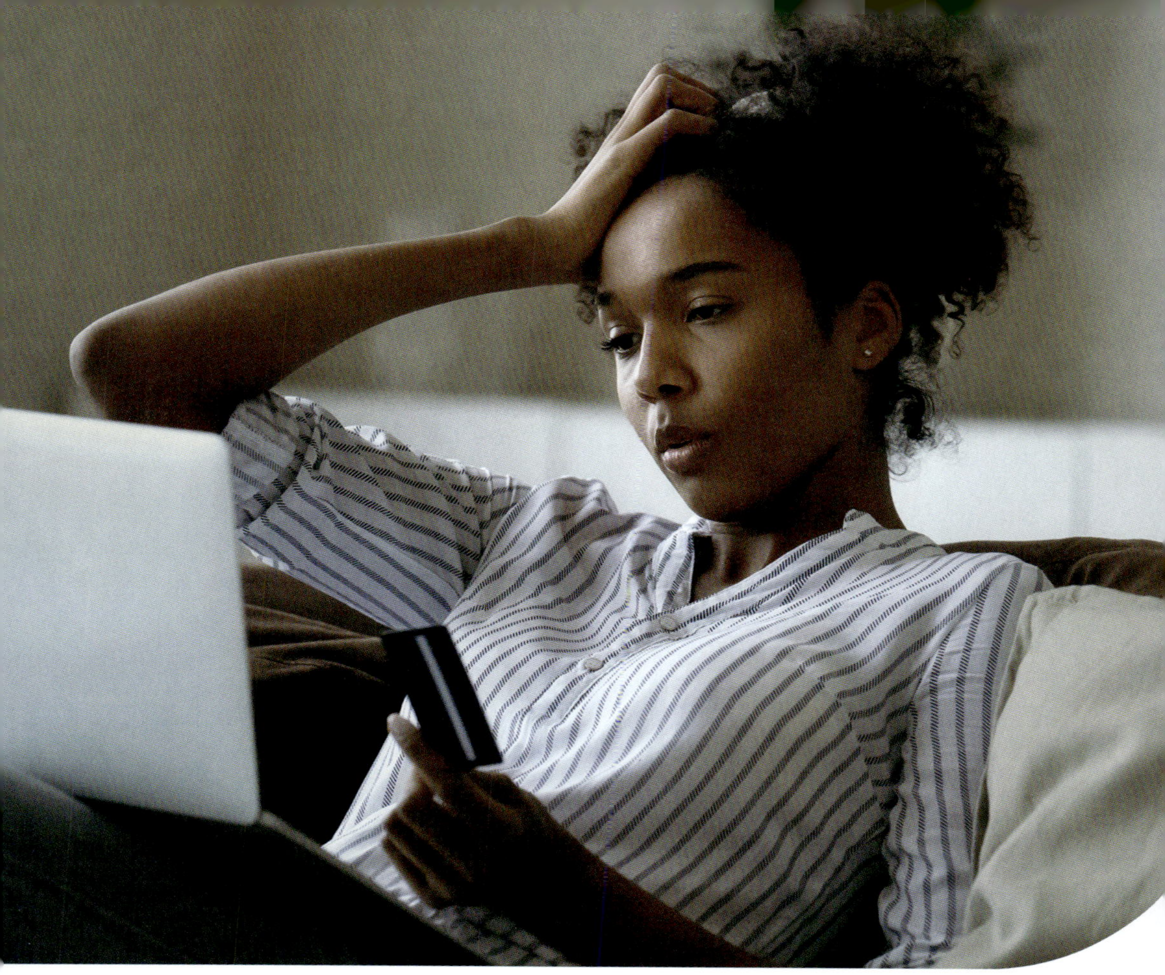

The rise of online gambling has made it easier for teenagers to develop gambling addictions.

Teens with mental disorders are especially more likely to develop addictions than their peers. According to the Child Mind Institute, nearly 50 percent of young people with mental disorders will develop an addiction if they do not receive

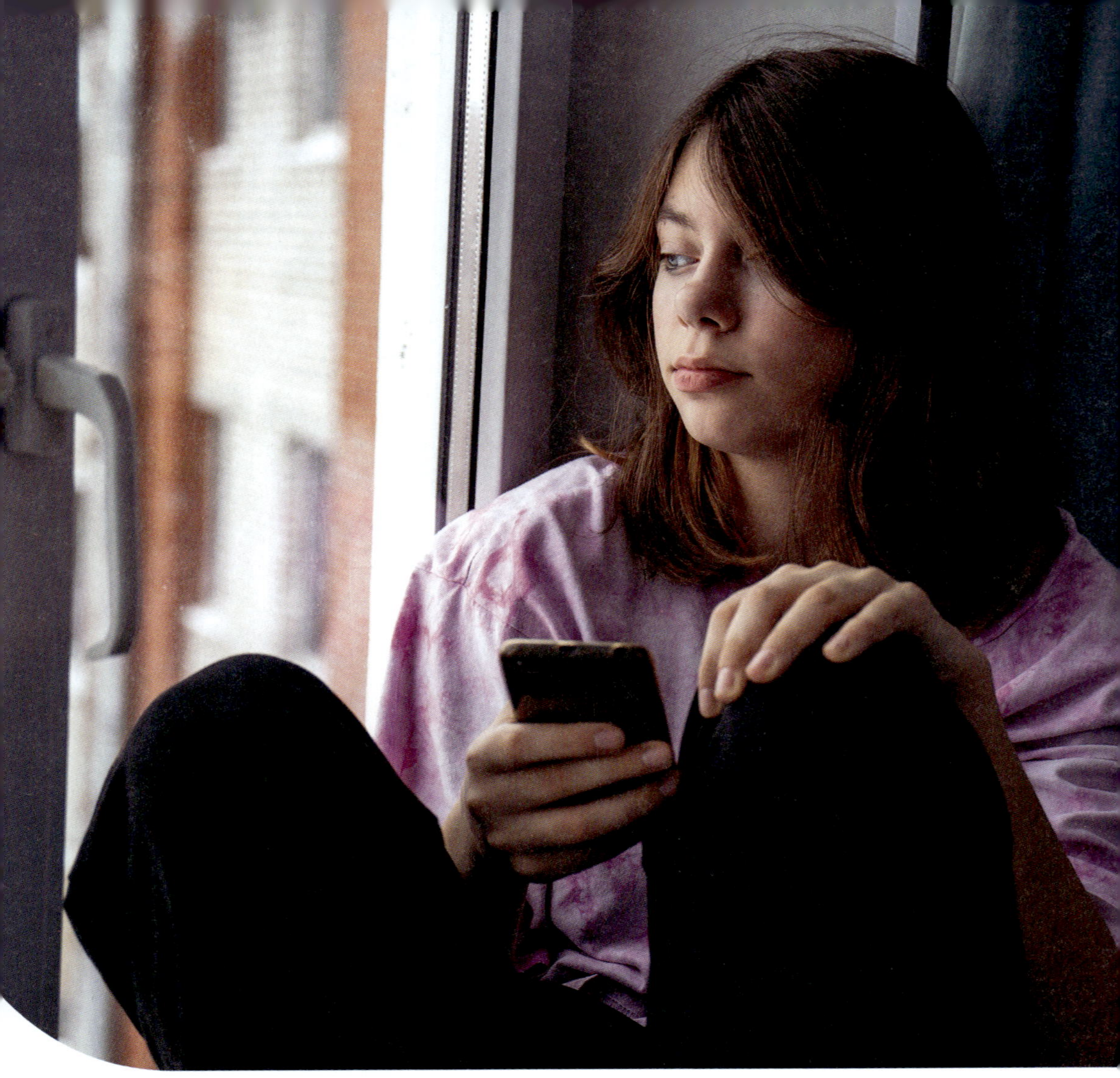



treatment for their mental illness. This

may be because mentally ill teens often

turn to drugs or addictive behaviors. They

use these activities to help them cope

with their problems. At first, drugs or behaviors may seem to help them manage their mental illnesses. But addictions can make these problems worse.

Brenden Tervo-Clemmens teaches psychiatry. He looked at data from more than 15,000 teens. The teens reported their substance use and mental health symptoms. Tervo-Clemmens found that "alcohol, **cannabis**, and nicotine use each had significant . . . associations with worse psychiatric symptoms, including suicidal thoughts." He added, "All the symptoms of mental health we examined, be it depression, suicidal thoughts, ADHD, were [worsened] no matter what the substance was."[5]

# CHAPTER TWO

# HOW ADDICTION AFFECTS TEENS

Addiction affects nearly all areas of life. It is particularly harmful to physical health. People who become addicted to smoking face high risks of many types of diseases. This includes cancer. And those with any drug addiction are at risk of overdosing. Overdosing can lead to brain damage. It can also lead to death.

Mental health is also affected by addiction. Some drugs make mental

**Smoking kills nearly half a million people in the United States each year.**

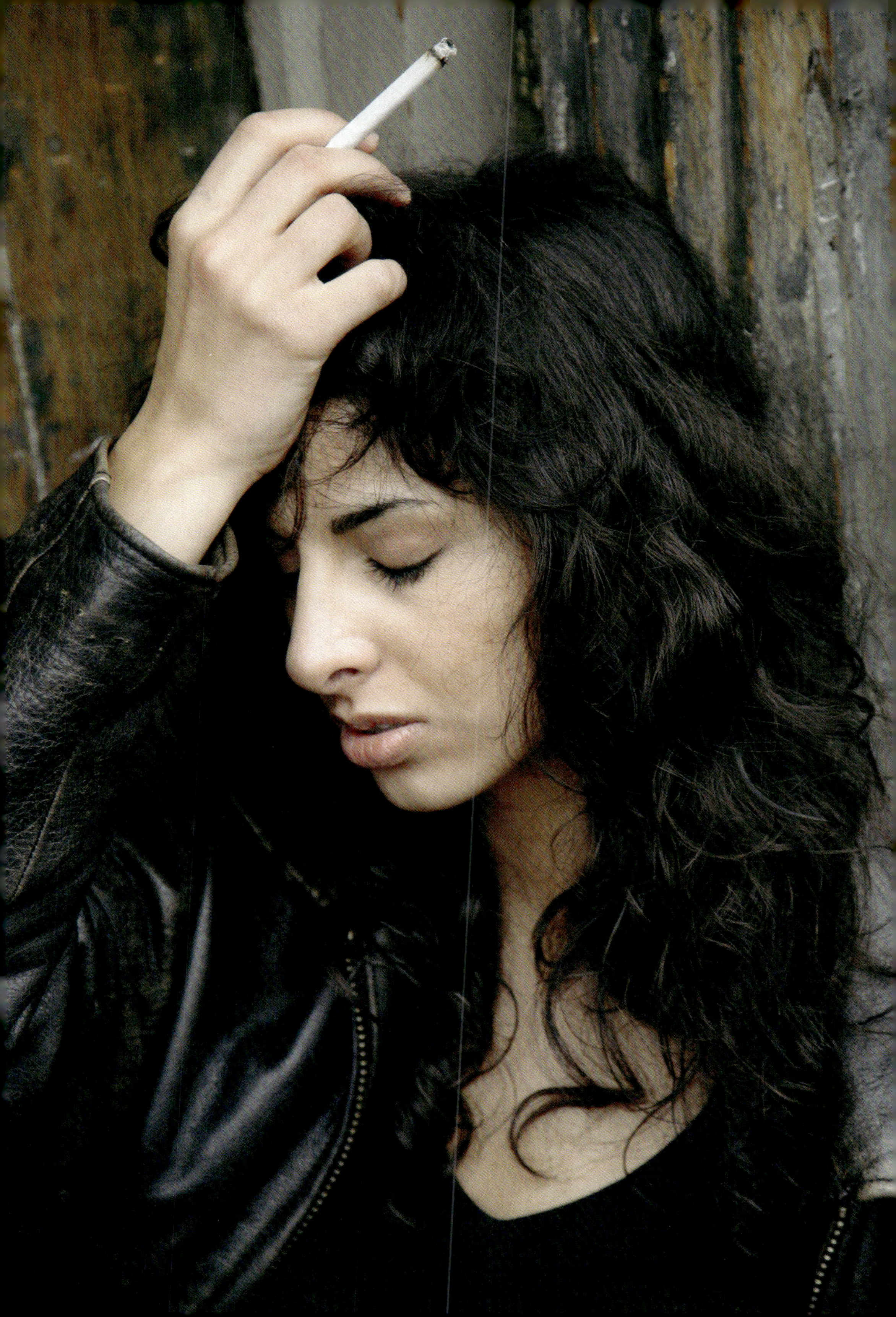

illnesses worse. Alcohol is one such drug. Dr. Akhil Anand says, "[Alcohol] can cause depression, worsen someone's depression, and can cause . . . anxiety."[6] Cocaine use can lead to anxiety or depression too.

**In 2021, more than 24,000 people in the United States died from cocaine overdoses.**

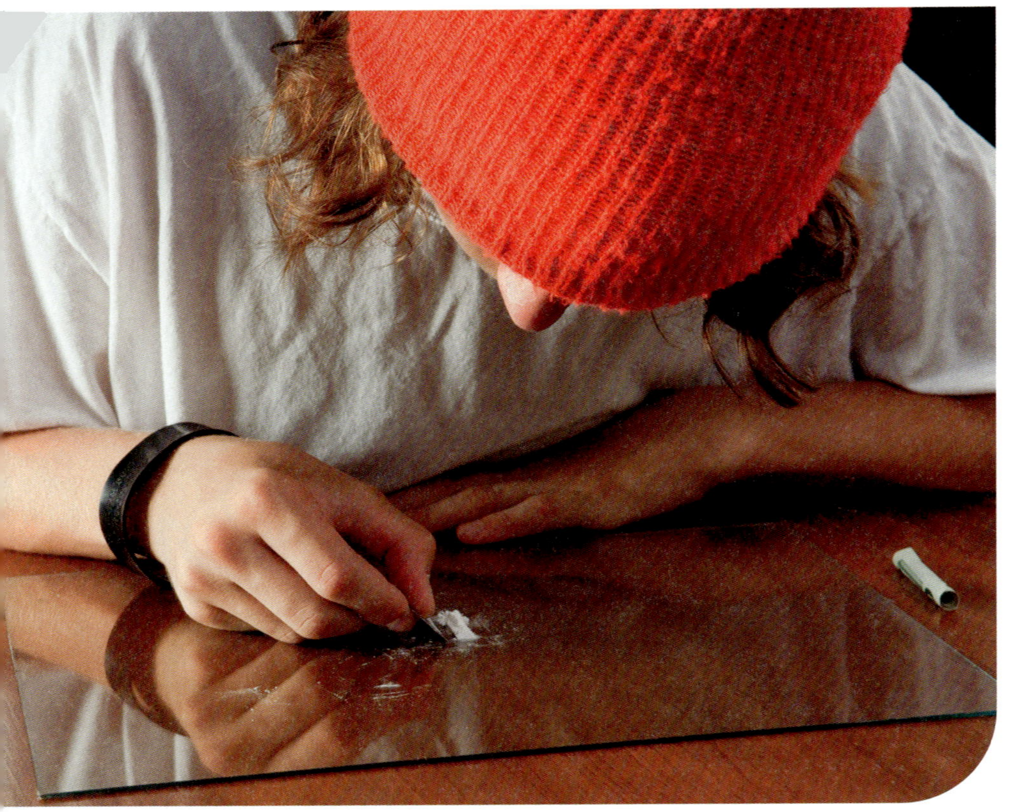

Some drugs can cause mental illnesses to develop faster. Excessive marijuana use has been linked to people developing schizophrenia earlier. **Methamphetamine** use has also been linked to schizophrenia. This disorder causes people to see or hear things that are not there. They may have a hard time thinking clearly.

## Overdosing

Overdosing is when a person takes a dangerous amount of a drug. It can also be caused by mixing drugs. Overdosing can have life-threatening consequences. In 2021, more than 1,000 adolescents died from drug overdoses. Signs of overdosing include confusion and vomiting. People may also pass out or have seizures. Emergency services should be called immediately if someone shows signs of overdosing.

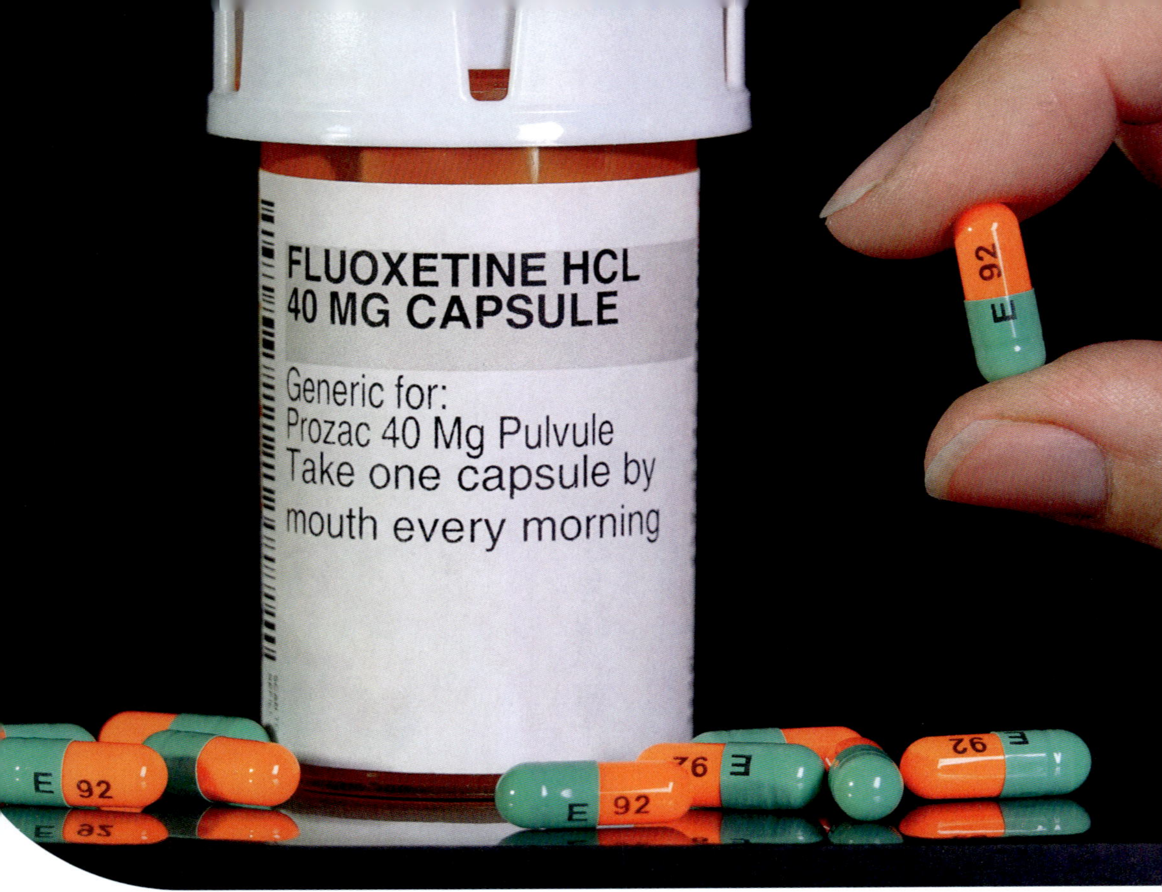


**Mixing alcohol with some antidepressants, such as fluoxetine, can lead to suicidal thoughts.**

Addictions can also get in the way of mental health treatment. They stop people from giving therapy their full attention. This stops them from fully benefiting from it.

Some drugs can make mental health medications less effective. Others can cause dangerous side effects. For example,

drinking alcohol while taking some
antidepressants can make people tired. It
can also cause high blood pressure. Using
marijuana while taking antidepressants can
cause heart problems. It may also make
people see things that are not there. It is
important to talk to a doctor before mixing
drugs and medications.

Other areas of a person's life may also
suffer due to addiction. Relationships
usually become strained. Some
relationships may be lost completely.
A person's education may also suffer.
Addiction can make it hard to go to school.
It can also make it hard to concentrate on
homework. People with addictions are more
likely to drop out of school. Those who work
may lose their jobs. Some people may even

get into legal trouble. They may be arrested
for having drugs. Others are arrested due to
their behavior under the influence of drugs.

## MICHAEL'S ALCOHOL ADDICTION

Michael King was bullied in school.
He often felt anxious and lonely. He
began drinking alcohol to cope with his
feelings. Drinking made him feel more
confident about himself. Alcohol made him
feel better when bad things happened. It
helped him celebrate when good things
happened. These habits led him to develop
an alcohol addiction in middle school.

Michael kept his drinking a secret. He
was under 21. This means it was illegal
for him to buy alcohol. He got alcohol by
shoplifting. He brought it home. Then he

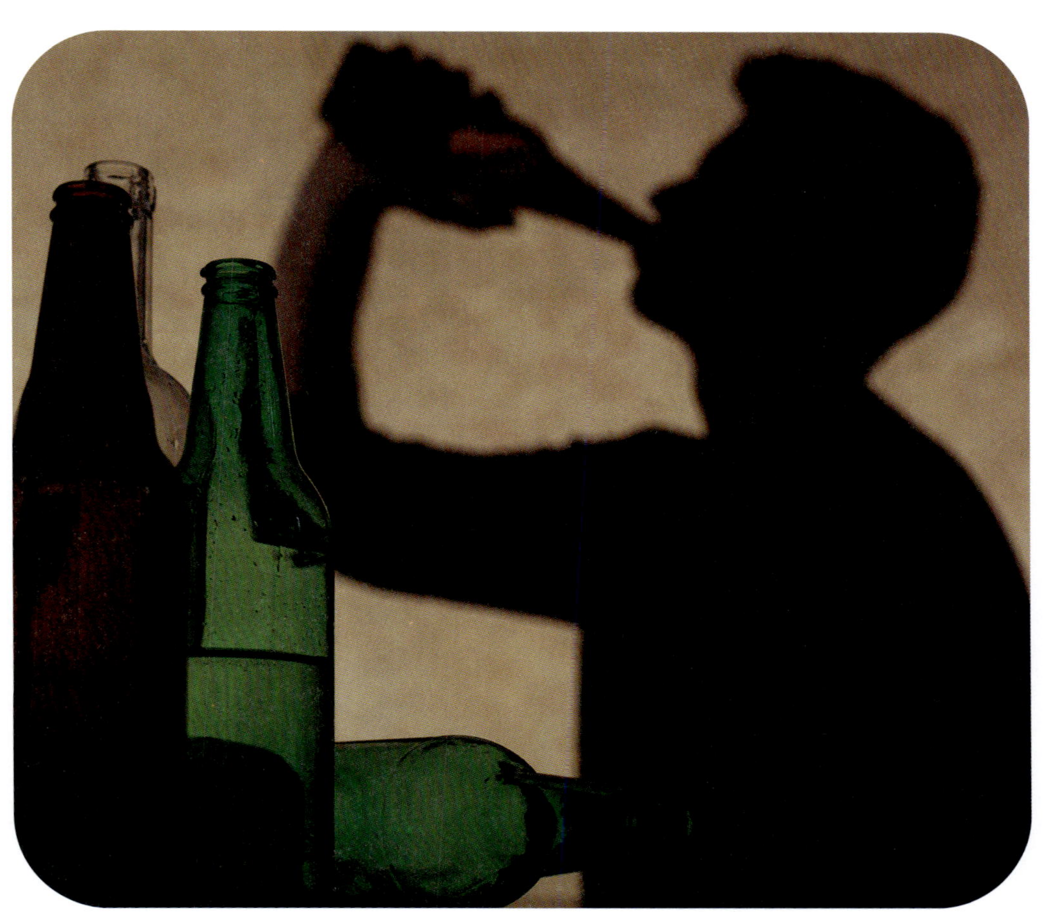

Victims of bullying are more likely to abuse alcohol than their peers.

drank it alone. He did not want his family members to discover his addiction.

Michael was 15 when he realized that he needed help. He wanted to stop drinking. He tried to recover. He stayed **sober** for more than 5 years. But he started

to feel jealous. He was upset that his
friends could drink while he could not.
His twenty-first birthday was getting closer.
He decided he would drink to celebrate. He
hoped he could handle it. He had a drink
2 days before his birthday. His addiction
once again spiraled out of control.

King spent the next 10 years drinking
every day. He recalls, "What had started
as a nightly ritual of a few beers turned
into . . . waking up to several shots of
whiskey in my coffee, drinking beer all day,
and ending with more hard alcohol and
marijuana at night."[7] King began gambling
too. He eventually ran out of money to
pay for alcohol. He began stealing money
from his employer. He needed it to fund
his addiction.

# TELE'S OPIOID ADDICTION

Tele was a happy and outgoing boy. He earned good grades. He played sports. He was popular. Tele and his friends started

**Tele (pictured) told his story to the Centers for Disease Control and Prevention to help others who are struggling with addiction.**

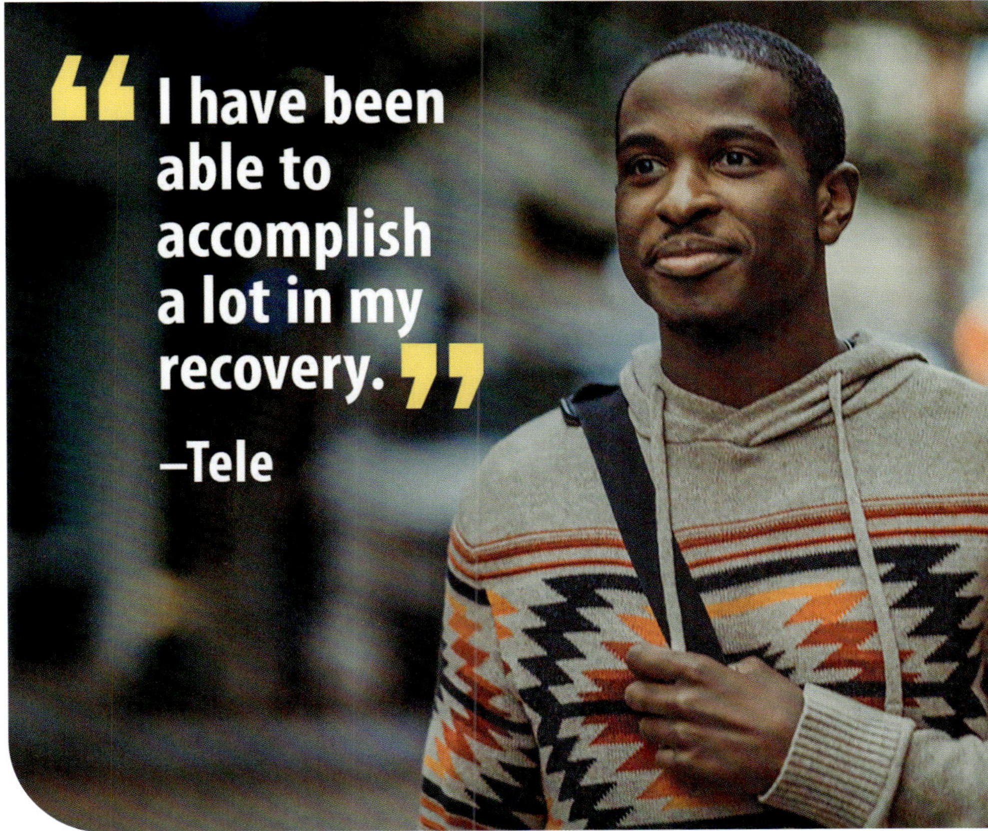

using prescription drugs at age 13. These are drugs that are given to someone by a doctor. Tele and his friends bought them illegally. Tele enjoyed the numbing effects of **opioids**.

**Doctors prescribe opioids to patients as painkillers.**

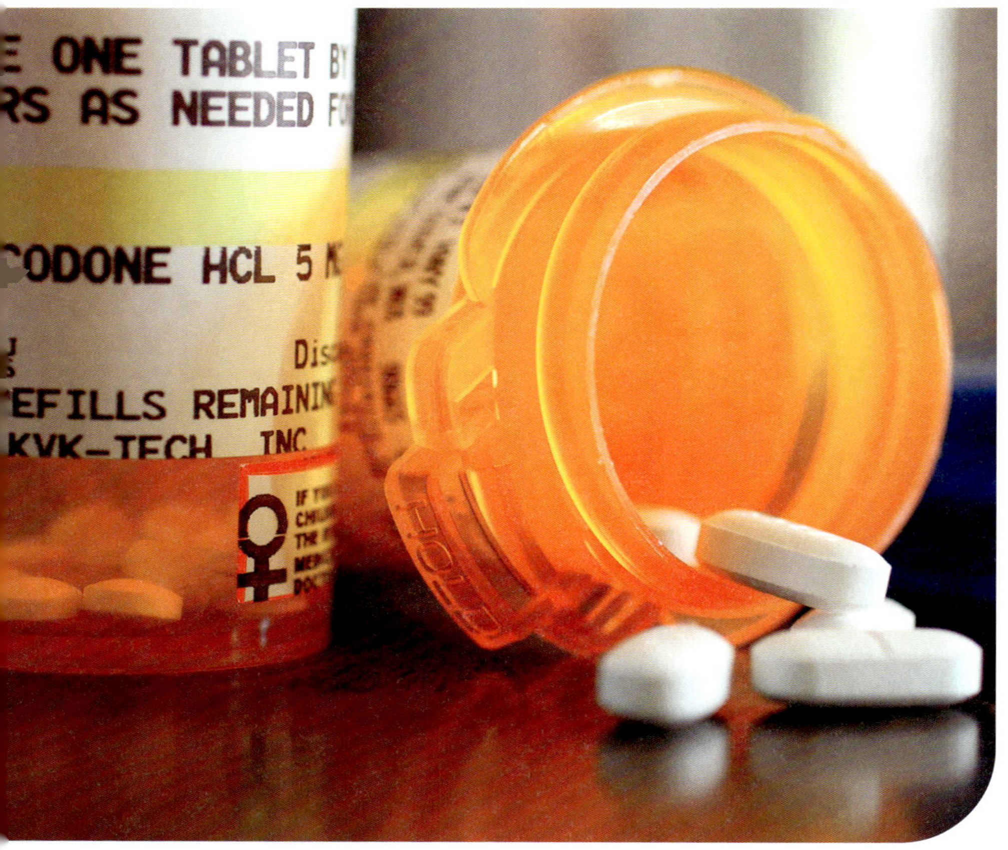

Tele began to feel alone as he got older. He had a lot of friends. But he was afraid to talk to them about his sexuality. He started using drugs more often to cope with his feelings.

Tele did not think that prescription pills could hurt him. He remembers thinking, "'They're medications. . . . They can't be that dangerous.'"[8]

Opioids soon became a part of Tele's everyday life. He did not realize that he was addicted. His body eventually grew used to the drugs. Prescription medications no longer gave him the high that he wanted. Tele started taking heroin instead. This opioid is powerful and illegal. Heroin can make it difficult for people to think or react quickly. It is also deadly.

Tele's world came crashing down the day he drove after taking heroin. He got into an accident. Police responded to the crash. They realized that Tele had been driving under the influence of drugs. Tele was arrested.

## STEVE'S GAMBLING ADDICTION

During an interview with *ABC News*, an 18-year-old man spoke about his gambling addiction. The man asked to be called Steve. He started gambling when he was 15 years old. He played a game called dice. He won a couple hundred dollars. It was thrilling. He wanted to gamble more.

Steve loved basketball and baseball. He played both games. He started betting on professional sports games. Steve was

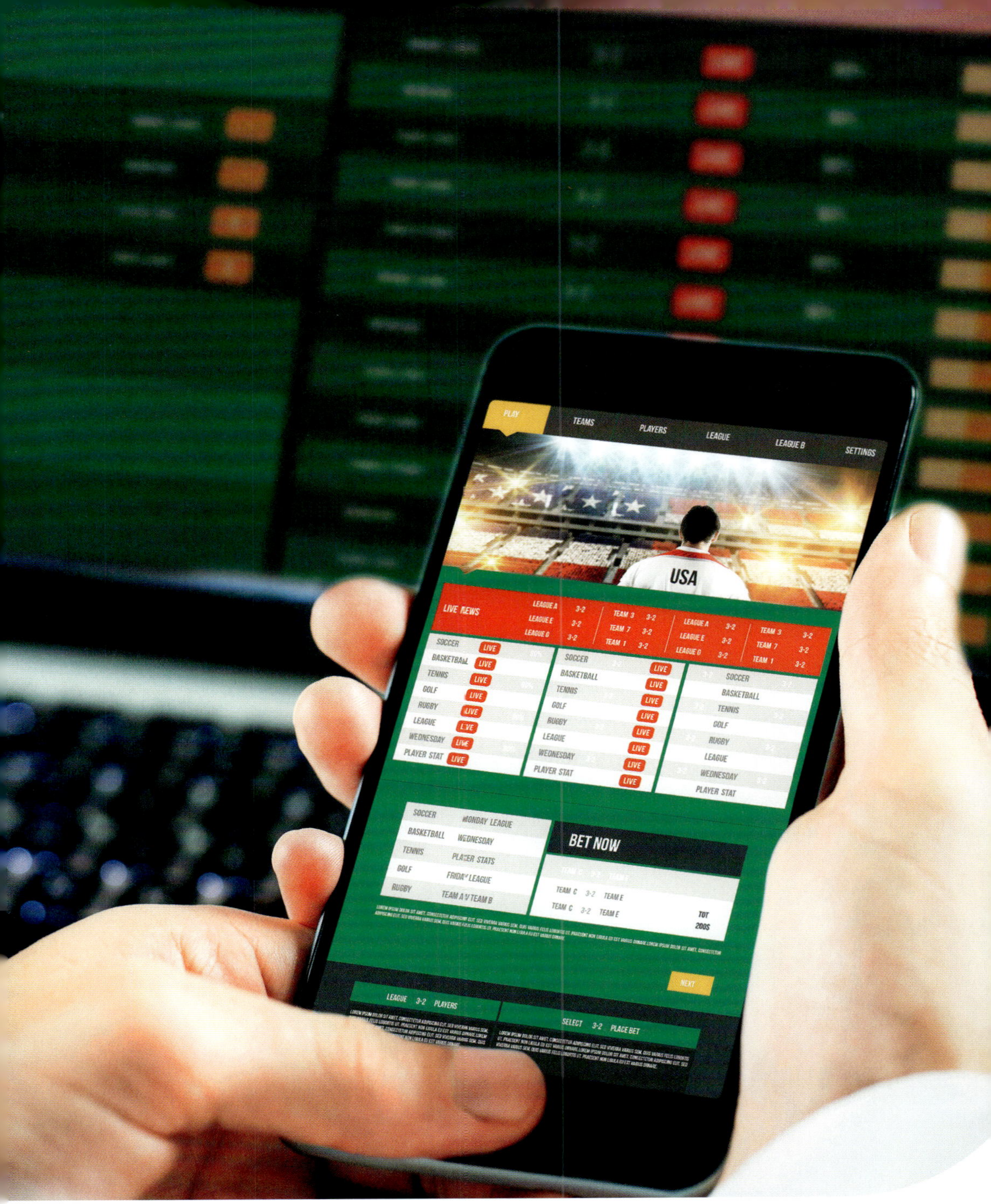

In 2022, Americans spent more than $93 billion on legal sports gambling.

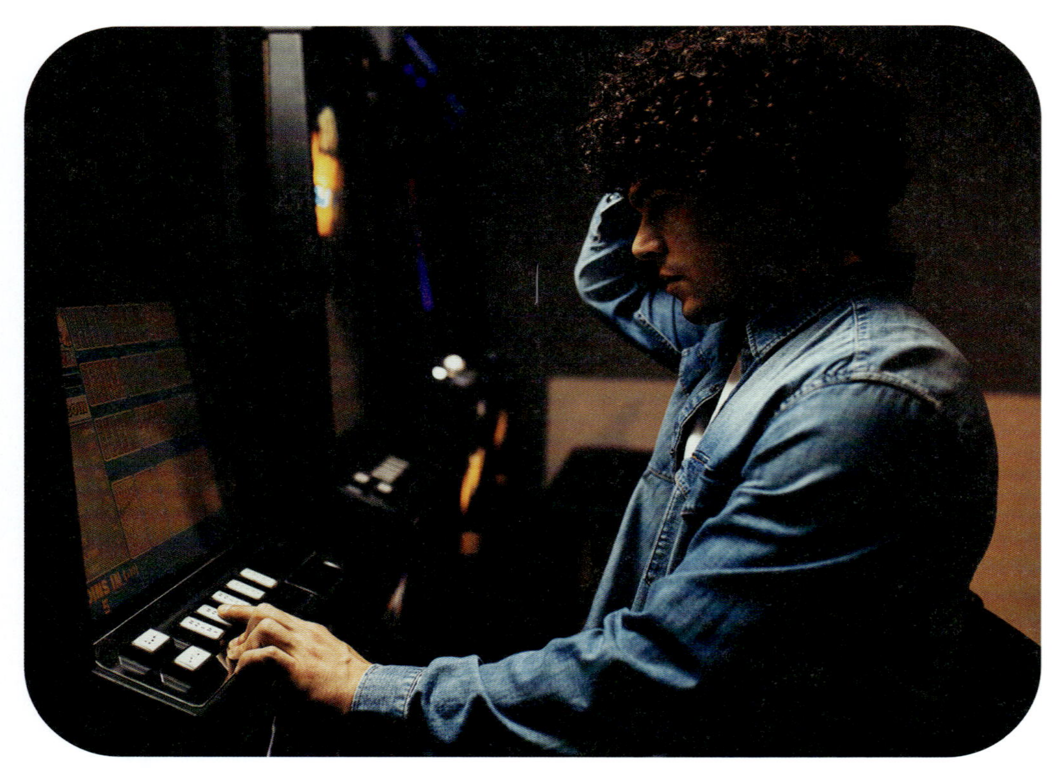

**People addicted to gambling have higher suicide rates than those with any other form of addiction.**

not old enough to bet on games legally. Most states require people to be at least 18 to gamble. Some states require people to be 21. Other states outlaw the practice entirely. But Steve wanted to gamble anyway. He used accounts belonging to his older friends. He also found illegal betting websites online.

Gambling was exciting. He began gambling whenever he was sad. He says, "I kind of used gambling as an escape from simple things like boredom, sadness, anger, even joy. Just like . . . drugs and alcohol for some people."[9]

Steve's gambling problem kept growing. Soon he was thousands of dollars in debt. But he could not stop. He started stealing money to be able to afford his addiction.

Addiction can change people's lives. The disorder may make people feel ashamed or scared. But addiction does not have to control people's lives forever. Recovery is possible. The first step is seeking help.

# CHAPTER THREE

# FINDING SUPPORT FOR ADDICTION

Many people with addictions do not realize they have a problem until something serious happens. Michael King realized he needed help when he ran out of money. He tried to steal more. But he could not find enough. He finally asked his family for support. They helped him find treatment. King went to a recovery center in Washington. He says, "Treatment forced me to see one thing crystal clear—my

**Many addiction treatment facilities are covered by health insurance.**

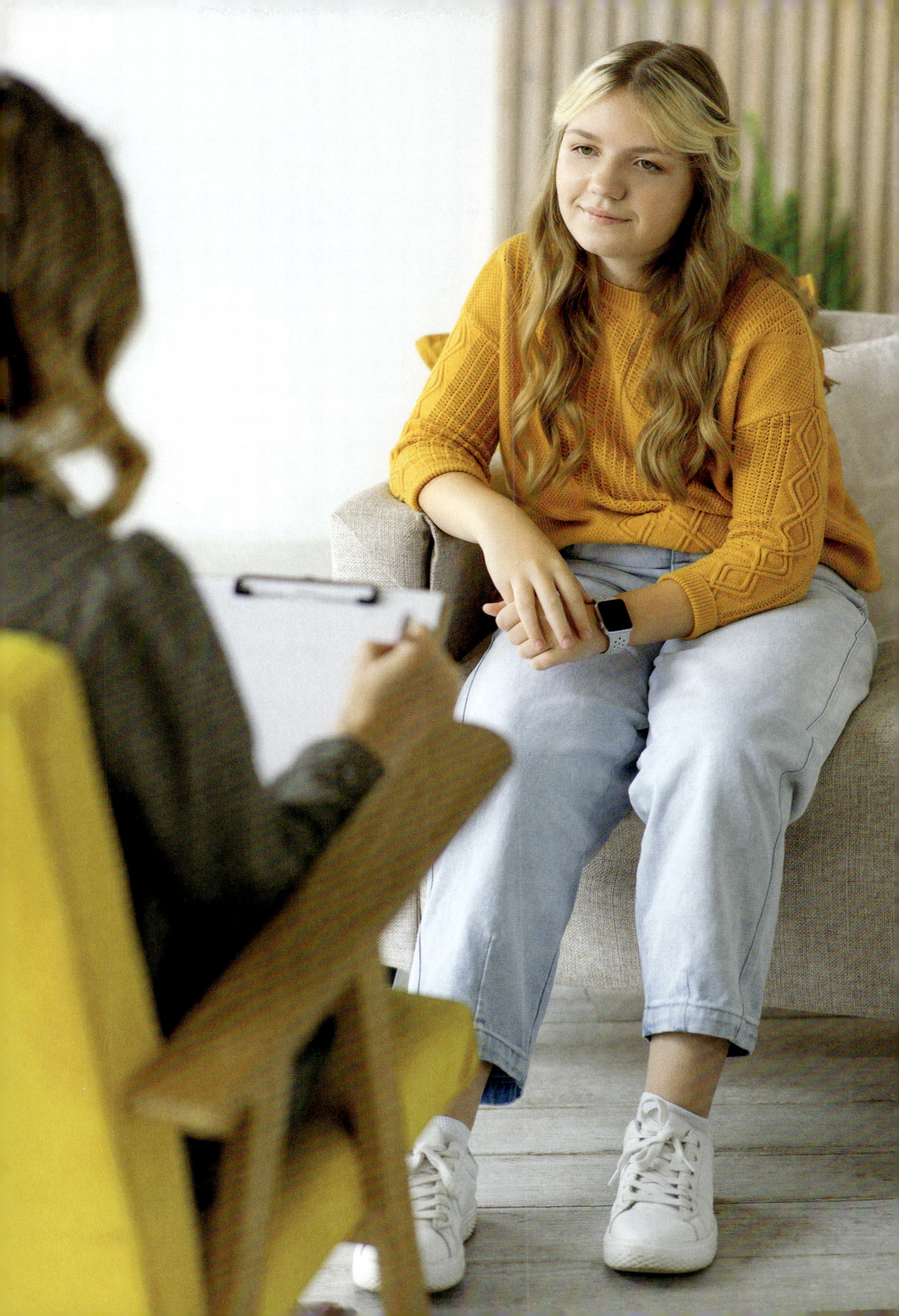

recovery had to be the most important thing in my life."[10] He is sure that treatment saved his life.

**When opening up about addiction, it is important to be honest.**

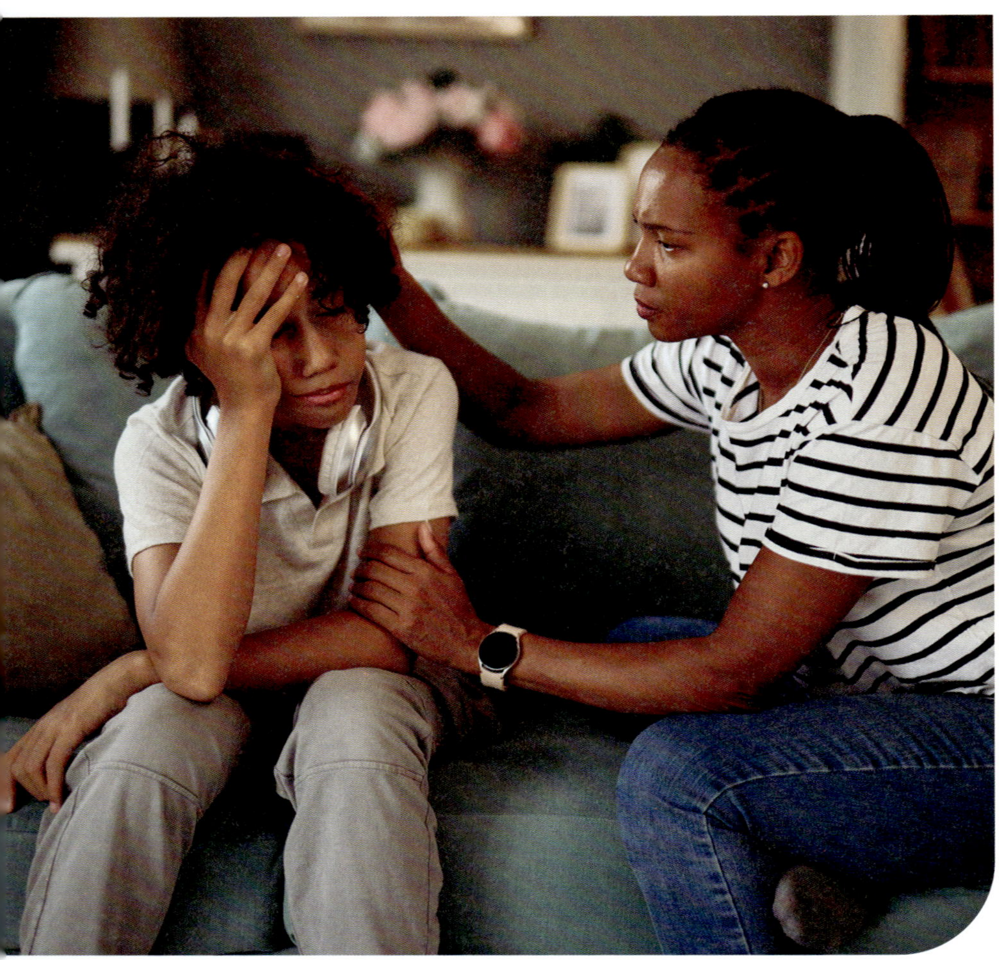

Tele did not realize that he needed help until he got arrested. He had thought he would not be able to have fun if he stopped taking opioids. He did not know how to live without drugs. But his parents helped him find treatment. So did his friends. They also supported him through recovery.

Steve continued gambling until his father discovered his problem. Steve lied to his parents about how much he was gambling. But they eventually realized how serious his addiction was. They helped him get treatment.

## FINDING HELP

People who think they may have an addiction often do not know how to get help. They can start by telling a loved one

about their problem. This person can offer
emotional support. The loved one can
help the addicted person find professional
treatment. People who have dealt with an
addiction can be especially helpful. They are
often willing to listen. They may even share
their own experiences. They know what it
is like to be at the start of this journey. They
can share what helped them most.

Many people are scared to tell others
about their addiction. They may worry about
being judged. Sometimes it can be easier
to tell someone about addiction in writing.
People can tell a friend or family member
through a letter or an email.

Teens struggling with addiction can reach
out to a teacher or school counselor. These
people are trained to help students navigate

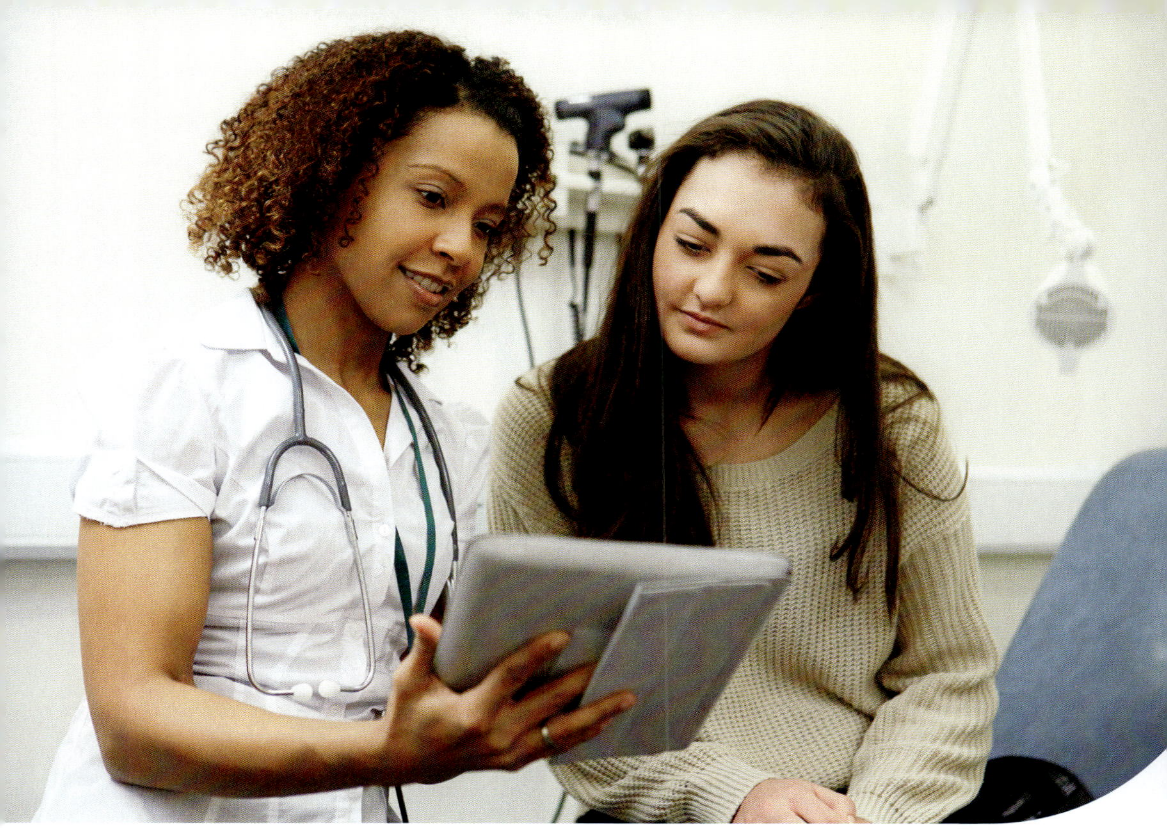

**Health care professionals do not disclose drug use to law enforcement.**

difficult situations. They can also connect students to support services.

The people who can help the most with addiction are health care professionals. These include doctors and therapists. These people can help patients reach out to someone who specializes in addiction treatment.

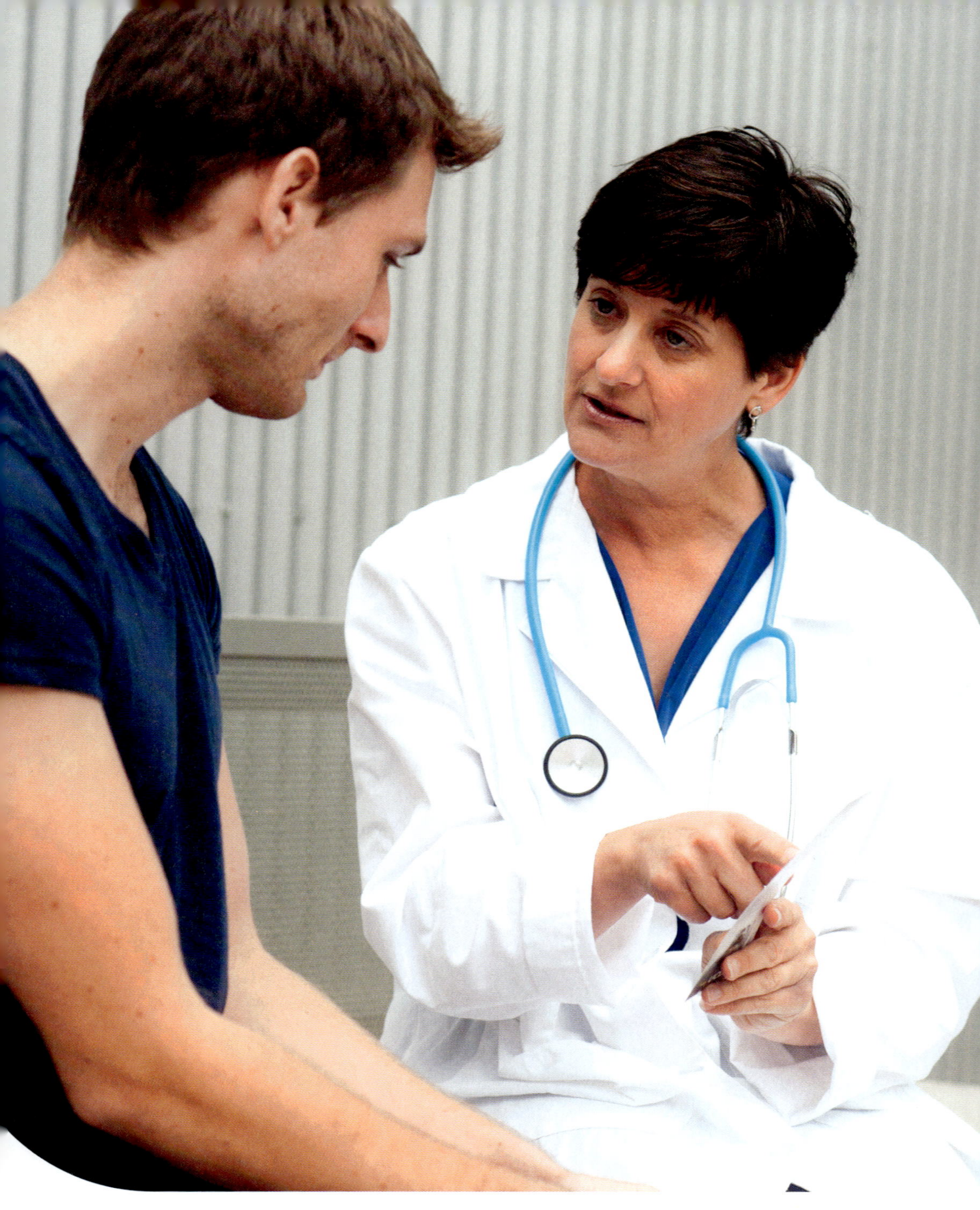

Alcohol withdrawal symptoms can begin as little as
6 hours after a person's last drink.

# GETTING TREATMENT

Addiction treatment typically begins with an assessment. The health care provider will ask the patient questions. The provider may discuss the person's addiction history. This conversation may be uncomfortable. But it will help the provider decide what treatment a person needs.

The first step of treatment for chemical addiction is detoxification. This is also called detox. Detox is the period when a drug leaves the body. Many people need help dealing with the withdrawal symptoms that happen during detox. Withdrawal symptoms are the body's reactions to stopping use of a drug. These symptoms can include mood swings. Withdrawal can also cause physical symptoms. These may include headaches and tremors. Doctors can provide medicine to help with these symptoms. The length of a detox varies for each person. It can take as long as 10 days.

People with behavioral addictions experience many of these same withdrawal symptoms. These symptoms can be just as severe as they are for people addicted to drugs. Medication can help manage these symptoms. Counseling can help as well.

It is important for detox to be done under a doctor's supervision. Withdrawal can be dangerous when a person's body is dependent on drugs. It can even be deadly. Patients need medicine to detox safely. Alcohol is one drug that people should not withdraw from without medical supervision. Without medicine, people may

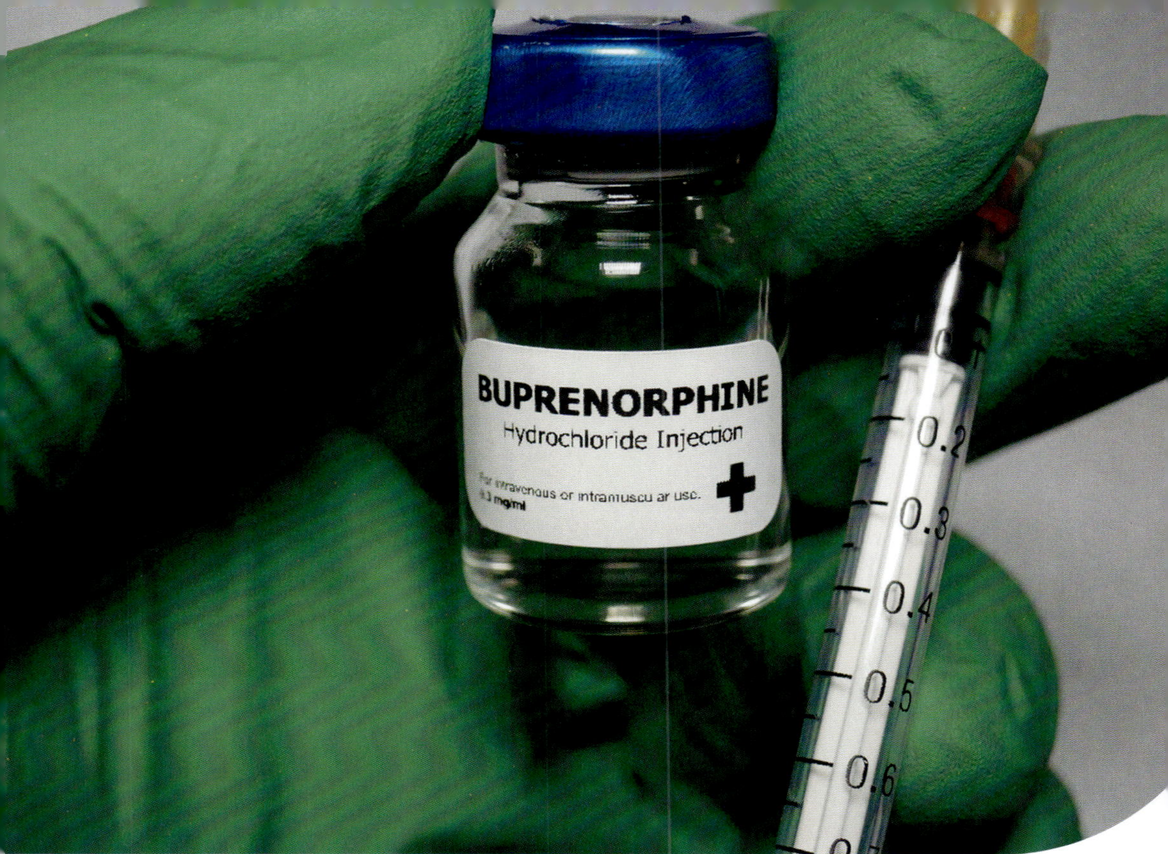


**Buprenorphine, also known as Suboxone, is one of the most common medications used to treat opioid withdrawal.**

have seizures. They may even die. This is especially true if the person has been heavily using alcohol for a long period of time.

Withdrawal from behavioral addictions can be dangerous too. People going through withdrawal may experience thoughts of suicide. Doctors can help manage these symptoms. They can also help patients avoid **relapsing**.

## TREATMENT PROGRAMS

Patients can move to the next step once detox has been completed. This step often involves a treatment program. There are several ways to receive treatment for addiction. One way is through outpatient treatment. The addicted person attends appointments with a therapist. The person goes home after each appointment. Outpatient treatment allows people to continue much of their daily routine. They can still go to school and work.

People may also receive inpatient treatment. People in inpatient care are admitted to a treatment center. They might stay there for weeks or months. Inpatient treatment centers allow people to receive medical attention at any time of the day. This can help people avoid relapsing. Inpatient care also allows people to devote more time to recovery.

## 12-Step Plan

Many people in treatment for addiction follow a 12-step plan. This common approach to addiction treatment was created in 1935. It was made to treat alcoholism. Today it is used to treat other types of addictions too. The first step requires patients to acknowledge their addictions. Other steps involve taking responsibility for any harm the addicted person has done.

Some people need more help than outpatient treatment provides. But they may not require an inpatient stay. These people may go to a partial hospitalization program. This type of treatment is often called day treatment because patients can go home each evening. Doctors can help patients figure out which type of care is best for them. Sometimes people start with inpatient treatment. Then they continue with partial hospitalization or outpatient treatment.

Some addiction treatment centers also offer help for mental illnesses. These places are called dual diagnosis treatment centers. They help people overcome addiction and mental illnesses at the same time. This can help prevent relapsing by addressing problems that can lead to addiction.

# THERAPY

Therapy is an important part of both inpatient and outpatient programs. There are several different types of therapy. Patients in treatment programs are often given individual therapy. This is one-on-one therapy with a counselor. Some people

**Before choosing a treatment facility, people should make sure the program is qualified.**

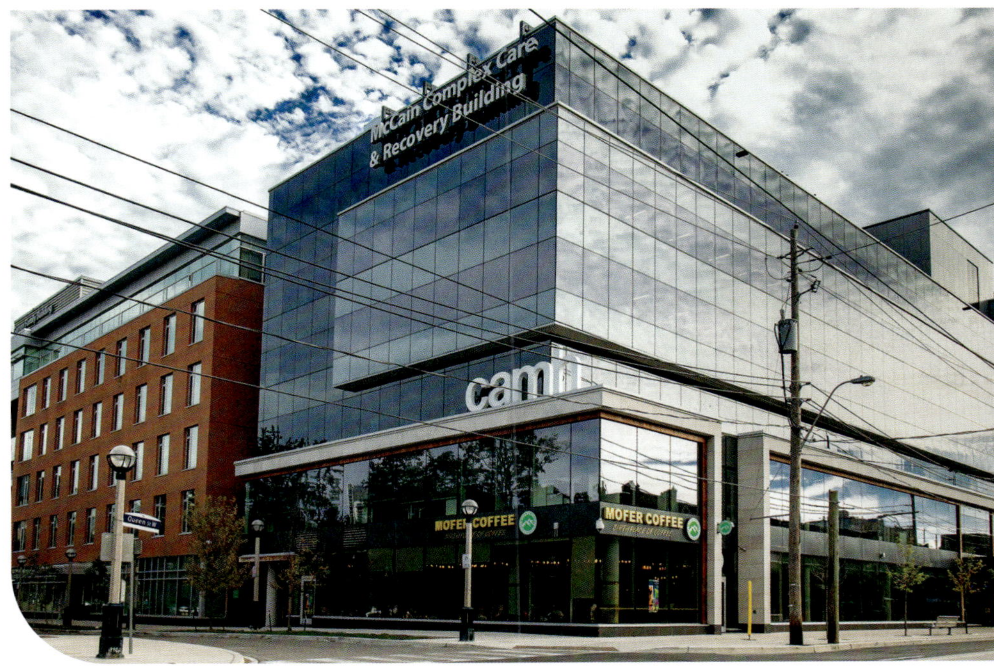

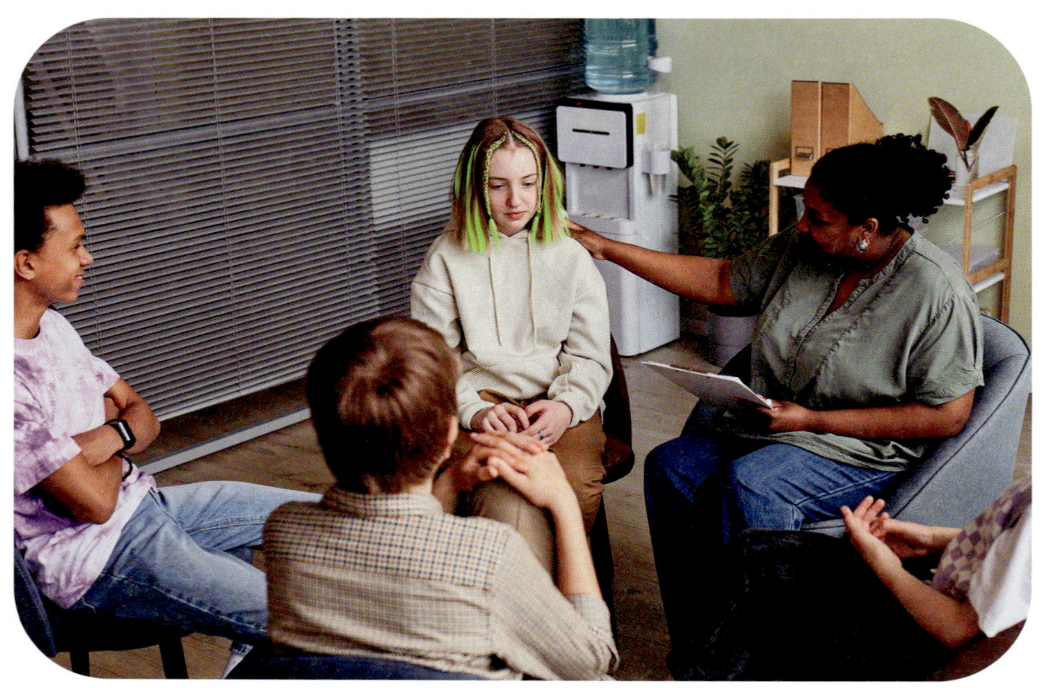

**Group therapy has been shown to be as effective as individual therapy at treating addiction.**

also receive family therapy. This involves sessions with a therapist for the patient and the patient's family. Other patients go to group therapy. This is a therapy session with a group of patients who have similar problems.

Therapists use different methods during sessions. Some practice cognitive behavioral therapy (CBT). This form of therapy teaches people to change negative thoughts and behaviors. Experts say CBT is one of the most effective treatments for addiction. Other therapists practice motivational interviewing. This form of therapy involves talking about addiction. It aims to increase the patient's desire to change the problem.

Recovering from addiction takes commitment and effort. It can be challenging. Up to 60 percent of people who receive treatment for drug addiction relapse. This is a normal part of recovery. People can return to treatment whenever they are ready to try again. The road to recovery is difficult. But people can overcome addiction. And no one needs to take the journey alone.

# GLOSSARY

**cannabis**

the plant that produces marijuana

**cocaine**

a highly addictive stimulant drug

**dopamine**

a chemical produced in the brain that makes people feel emotionally and physically good

**methamphetamine**

a strong, highly addictive stimulant drug

**opioids**

depressant drugs that produce numbness for pain relief

**relapsing**

returning to drug use after a period of sobriety

**sober**

not under the influence of drugs

**tremors**

trembling or unintentional movements

**vaping**

using an electronic cigarette to inhale vapor that usually contains nicotine

# SOURCE NOTES

### INTRODUCTION: ADDICTED TO VAPING

1. Luka Kinard and A. Pawlowski, "16-Year-Old Went to Rehab for Vaping Addiction," *Today*, September 16, 2019. www.today.com.

### CHAPTER ONE: WHAT IS ADDICTION?

2. Quoted in Amy Paturel, "How Do Video Games Affect Brain Development in Children and Teens?" *Brain & Life*, June/July 2014. www.brainandlife.org.

3. Quoted in Caroline Miller, "Mental Health Disorders and Teen Substance Use," *Child Mind Institute*, October 30, 2023. https://childmind.org.

4. Quoted in Allie Weintraub, Sarah Lang, and Stephanie Lorenzo, "Online Gambling Among Youth Worries Experts, One Teen Says Sports Betting Was an 'Escape,'" *ABC News*, December 8, 2022. https://abcnews.go.com.

5. Quoted in Matt Richtel, "Teen Drug and Alcohol Use Linked to Mental Health Distress," *New York Times*, January 29, 2024. www.nytimes.com.

### CHAPTER TWO: HOW ADDICTION AFFECTS TEENS

6. Quoted in "Dual Diagnosis: Why Substance Misuse Worsens Your Mental Health," *Cleveland Clinic*, May 23, 2021. https://health.clevelandclinic.org.

7. Michael King, "My Addiction Recovery Story," *Addiction Education Society*, n.d. https://addictioneducationsociety.org.

8. Quoted in "Tele's Rx Awareness Story," *YouTube*, uploaded by Centers for Disease Control and Prevention (CDC), July 10, 2020. www.youtube.com.

9. Quoted in Weintraub et al., "Online Gambling Among Youth Worries Experts."

### CHAPTER THREE: FINDING SUPPORT FOR ADDICTION

10. King, "My Addiction Recovery Story."

# FOR FURTHER RESEARCH

## BOOKS

Renae Gilles, *Understanding Drugs*. Ann Arbor, MI: Cherry Lake, 2020.

Elizabeth Hobbs Voss, *Vaping Addiction.* San Diego, CA: BrightPoint Press, 2023.

Philip Wolny, *Teens Dealing with Mental Illness*. San Diego, CA: BrightPoint Press, 2025.

## INTERNET SOURCES

"Find Help," *Get Smart About Drugs*, March 28, 2024. www.getsmartaboutdrugs.gov.

"Scientists Answer Addiction Questions from Teens," *Just Think Twice*, n.d. www.justthinktwice.gov.

Leah Walker, "Resources for Teens About Drug and Alcohol Abuse," *Project Know*, August 11, 2023. https://projectknow.com.

# WEBSITES

## The Centers for Disease Control
www.cdc.gov

The Centers for Disease Control and Prevention (CDC) was founded in 1946. Since its creation, the organization has been devoted to studying and preventing diseases both in the United States and around the world. Its "Health Topics A-Z" page contains links to pages about addiction.

## Mayo Clinic
www.mayoclinic.org

The Mayo Clinic is a nonprofit organization devoted to researching and treating medical conditions. Its "Diseases & Conditions" page contains links to pages about different types of addiction.

## Substance Abuse and Mental Health Services Administration
www.samhsa.gov

The Substance Abuse and Mental Health Services Administration (SAMHSA) was created to link people suffering from substance abuse disorders and mental illnesses with treatment services. Its free phone helpline offers resources 24/7 in both English and Spanish. Its website includes informative articles and resources to help people struggling with addiction.

12-step plan, 53

ABC News, 38
alcohol, 12–16, 17, 18, 25, 28, 31,
    32–34, 41, 50–51, 53
Anand, Akhil, 28

Center for Internet and Technology
    Addiction, 18
Child Mind Institute, 23
cigarettes, 14–15
cocaine, 7, 28

detoxification, 49–52

Fong, Timothy, 22
Friedman, Jeanette, 21–22

gambling, 10, 14, 18, 22, 34,
    38–41, 45
Greenfield, David, 18

heroin, 37–38

Kinard, Luka, 6–10
King, Michael, 32–34, 42–44

marijuana, 12, 15, 25, 29, 31, 34
mental illnesses, 23–25, 26–31, 54
methamphetamine, 29

opioids, 36–37, 45
overdosing, 26, 29

physical effects, 8, 10, 26, 29, 31,
    37, 49–51

recovery, 8, 41, 42–57
relapsing, 52–54, 57
reward system, 16–20

Steve, 38–41, 45

Tele, 35–38, 45
Tervo-Clemmens, Brenden, 25
therapy, 11, 30, 47, 52, 55–57
tolerance, 18
treatment centers, 8, 42, 52–54, 55

UCLA Gambling Studies
    Program, 22

vaping, 6–10
video games, 18–20

withdrawal, 49–52

# IMAGE CREDITS

Cover: © filadendron/iStockphoto

5: © Motortion Films/Shutterstock Images

7: © Mariia Masich/Shutterstock Images

9: © Monkey Business Images/Shutterstock Images

11: © SeventyFour/iStockphoto

13: © Sabphoto/Shutterstock Images

15: © Red Line Editorial

16: © zizou7/Shutterstock Images

19: © RicardoImagen/iStockphoto

21: © pixfly/Shutterstock Images

23: © fizkes/iStockphoto

24: © Andrey Znamenskyi/iStockphoto

27: © John Sommer/iStockphoto

28: © threerocksimages/Shutterstock Images

30: © Simone Hogan/Shutterstock Images

33: © KatarzynaBialasiewicz/iStockphoto

35: © CDC

36: © Peter Kim/Shutterstock Images

39: © Wavebreak Media/Shutterstock Images

40: © skynesher/iStockphoto

43: © spb2015/iStockphoto

44: © stockphotodirectors/iStockphoto

47: © Monkey Business Images/iStockphoto

48: © pkchai/Shutterstock Images

51: © Hailshadow/iStockphoto

55: © sockagphoto/Shutterstock Images

56: © SeventyFour/Shutterstock Images

# ABOUT THE AUTHOR

Tammy Gagne is an author and editor who specializes in nonfiction. She has written hundreds of books for both children and adults. She lives in northern New England with her husband, son, and dogs.